Type 2 Diabetes

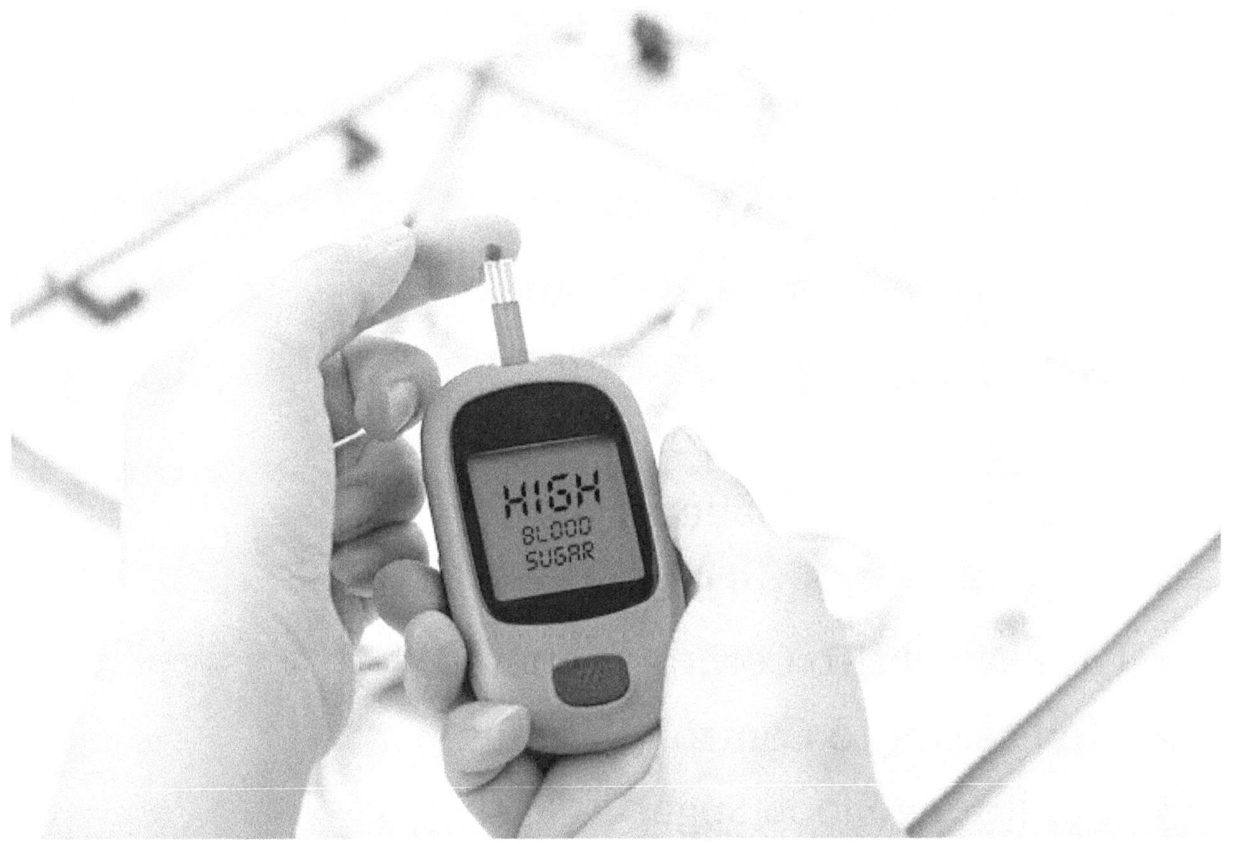

How To Get Freedom From Diabetes & Control Blood Sugar Level?

Table of Contents –

- What is Type 2 Diabetes?
- When Type 2 Diabetes Occur?
- How Diabetes is Diagnose?
- How To Control Diabetes?
- Diet To Control Diabetes
- Exercise To Control Diabetes
- Lose Weight To Control Diabetes
- Medication To Control Diabetes
- Monitoring Blood Sugar
- Bariatric Surgery
- Diabetes Complications To Watch Out For
- Conclusion

What is Type 2 Diabetes?

Type 2 diabetes is the predominant form of diabetes, impacting approximately 90% of the over 30 million Americans diagnosed with diabetes. Unlike type 1 diabetes, which results from an autoimmune response attacking insulin-producing cells, type 2 diabetes is often associated with lifestyle factors. In this condition, the body either fails to effectively use insulin or the cells develop resistance to it, leading to elevated blood sugar levels. While it cannot be cured, type 2 diabetes is manageable through a comprehensive approach involving lifestyle modifications, including diet and exercise, and, when necessary, the incorporation of medications.

In essence, type 2 diabetes involves a disruption in the body's ability to regulate blood sugar levels, and its prevalence underscores the significance of lifestyle factors in its development. The condition necessitates ongoing management to prevent complications and improve overall health.

When Type 2 Diabetes Occur?

Type 2 diabetes typically arises within a broader context of health, often manifesting after a phase known as prediabetes. Prediabetes is characterized by elevated blood sugar levels that are not yet in the diabetic range. The risk factors for both prediabetes and type 2 diabetes are multifaceted and include lifestyle elements as well as genetic predispositions.

The onset of type 2 diabetes is associated with factors such as being overweight or obese, having a family history of diabetes, and leading a sedentary lifestyle. Individuals aged 45 or older are at a higher risk, and those with a history of gestational diabetes or who have given birth to a baby over 9 pounds may also be more susceptible. Moreover, belonging to certain ethnic groups, including African American, Hispanic, American Indian, Alaska Native, Pacific Island, or Asian American descent, increases the likelihood of developing type 2 diabetes.

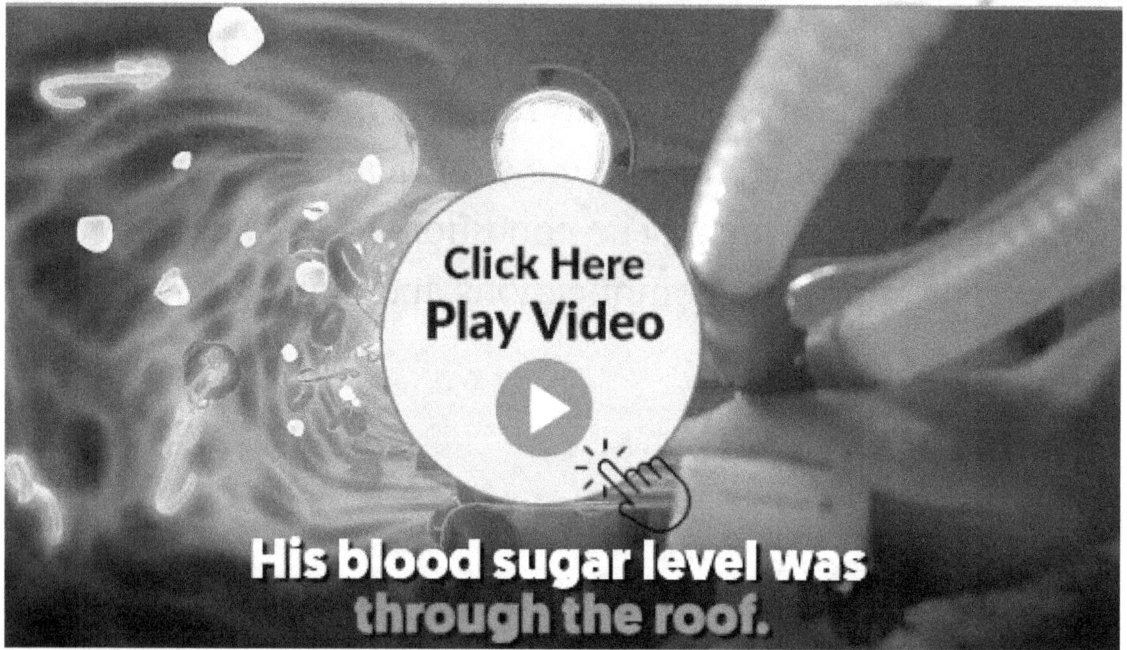

<u>Watch: How Diabetes Can Become Dangerous?</u>

While age is a contributing factor, it's noteworthy that diabetes doesn't discriminate by age, and even children can be diagnosed with type 2 diabetes, especially as childhood obesity rates have risen. The number of youths with type 2 diabetes is still relatively small, but as childhood obesity becomes more prevalent, these numbers are expected to increase.

In essence, the occurrence of type 2 diabetes is intricately linked to a combination of genetic, lifestyle, and environmental factors, making it imperative to recognize the risk factors and take preventive measures, particularly through healthy lifestyle choices.

How Diabetes is Diagnose?

Diagnosing diabetes, particularly type 2 diabetes, involves a series of tests designed to measure blood sugar levels and identify the presence of the condition. Given that early-stage type 2 diabetes may not exhibit noticeable symptoms, regular screenings are vital, especially for individuals with risk factors. The diagnostic process encompasses various tests and considerations.

1. Blood Sugar Tests:

   - A1C Test: This common test measures glycated hemoglobin (A1C), providing an average blood sugar level over the past two to three months. An A1C level of 6.5% on two separate tests indicates diabetes, while levels between 5.7% and 6.4% suggest prediabetes.

- **Fasting Blood Sugar Test:** This test measures blood sugar levels after an overnight fast. A fasting blood sugar level of 126 milligrams per deciliter (mg/dL) or higher indicates diabetes.

2. Oral Glucose Tolerance Test (OGTT):

- This test involves fasting overnight, followed by drinking a sugary solution. Blood sugar levels are then tested periodically over the next few hours. A blood sugar level of 200 mg/dL or higher two hours after drinking the solution indicates diabetes.

3. Random Blood Sugar Test:

- This test involves checking blood sugar levels at any time, regardless of when the individual last ate. A blood sugar level of 200 mg/dL or higher, along with symptoms of diabetes, may suggest the condition.

4. Additional Considerations for Testing:

- Individuals with risk factors, such as being overweight, having a family history of diabetes, or having a history of gestational diabetes, may undergo routine blood sugar tests during annual check-ups.

- Urine tests for specific byproducts may be recommended if there's suspicion of type 1 diabetes rather than type 2.

It's crucial for individuals with risk factors to initiate a dialogue with their healthcare providers about routine diabetes screening.

Early detection is key, especially since symptoms may be mild or absent in the early stages. Understanding one's risk factors and engaging in proactive testing are fundamental components of the diagnostic process. Regular check-ups, particularly for those with risk factors, contribute to the timely identification and management of diabetes.

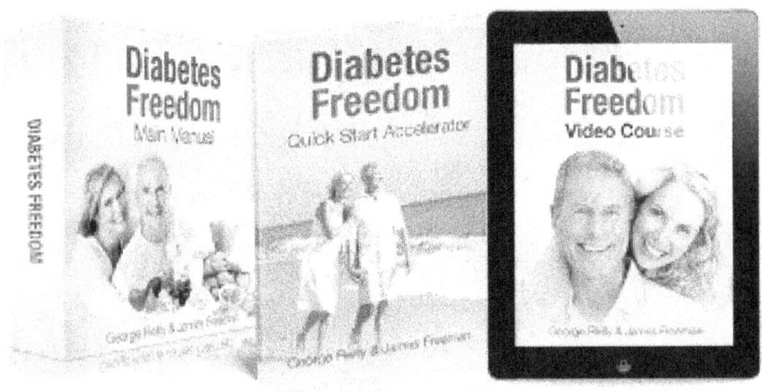

[Click Here To Get Freedom From Diabetes](#)

How To Control Diabetes?

Controlling diabetes involves a multifaceted approach, empowering individuals to actively manage their blood sugar levels and mitigate potential complications. The comprehensive strategy encompasses lifestyle changes, medication management, and vigilant monitoring. Here's a detailed exploration of how to control diabetes:

1. Education and Awareness:

   - Begin by acquiring a deep understanding of diabetes management. Seek guidance from healthcare professionals, including certified diabetes educators, dietitians, or participation in diabetes education programs.

2. Lifestyle Changes:

- **Dietary Modifications:** Adopting a balanced diet is paramount. Emphasize whole foods, including fruits, vegetables, whole grains, lean proteins, and healthy fats. Limit the intake of sugary foods, saturated fats, and high-sodium items. Collaborate with a dietitian to tailor dietary changes to individual preferences and health needs.

- **Physical Activity:** Regular exercise is instrumental in managing blood sugar levels. Aim for at least 150 minutes of brisk movement per week, including aerobic activities and strength training. Even brief, regular bursts of activity yield significant health benefits.

3. Weight Management:

- For those who are overweight or obese, gradual and sustainable weight loss can significantly improve blood sugar control. Consulting with healthcare professionals helps formulate safe and personalized weight loss plans.

4. Medication Management:

- Medications may be prescribed to lower glucose production, increase insulin sensitivity, or enhance insulin production. Some individuals may require insulin therapy. Collaborate with healthcare providers to determine the most suitable medication plan, recognizing that medication needs may evolve over time.

5. Monitoring Blood Sugar Levels:

- Regularly monitor blood sugar levels to understand how lifestyle changes and medications impact glycemic control. Utilize glucose meters to measure levels, adhering to recommended targets provided by healthcare providers.

6. Bariatric Surgery:

- In cases where traditional weight management methods are challenging, bariatric surgery may be considered, particularly for individuals with a body mass index (BMI) over 35. It's crucial to weigh the potential benefits against the risks and commit to lifelong lifestyle changes.

7. Diabetes Complications Prevention:

- Proactively address potential complications associated with diabetes, such as vision problems, slow-healing wounds, and cardiovascular issues. Regular eye exams, foot care, and cardiovascular health management contribute to prevention.

8. Regular Follow-ups:

- Stay connected with healthcare providers for regular check-ups. Diabetes management is dynamic, and adjustments to lifestyle and medication plans may be necessary. Regular follow-ups ensure that the current approach aligns with individual health needs.

9. Continuous Self-Management:

- Empower individuals to take an active role in their diabetes management. By combining education, lifestyle changes, medication adherence, and ongoing monitoring, individuals can gain control over their condition and work towards achieving optimal blood sugar levels.

In conclusion, controlling diabetes is a collaborative effort that involves informed decision-making, lifestyle adjustments, medication management, and regular monitoring. It's a dynamic process that requires ongoing commitment and adaptation to individual needs. By embracing a comprehensive approach, individuals with diabetes can enhance their overall well-being and minimize the risk of complications.

Diet To Control Diabetes –

Managing diabetes through a well-crafted diet is a cornerstone of effective diabetes control. Here's an in-depth exploration of the dietary principles that contribute to controlling diabetes:

1. Personalized Approach:

- Recognize that there's no one-size-fits-all diet for diabetes. Collaborate with healthcare professionals, particularly dietitians, to develop a personalized dietary plan tailored to individual preferences, lifestyle, and medical needs.

2. Emphasis on Whole Foods:

- Prioritize whole, nutrient-dense foods. Incorporate a variety of fruits and vegetables rich in fiber, vitamins, and minerals. These foods contribute to overall health and help manage blood sugar levels.

3. Carbohydrate Management:

- Carbohydrates directly influence blood sugar levels. Monitor and control carbohydrate intake, especially from refined sources. Choose complex carbohydrates like whole grains, oats, brown rice, and legumes, which have a slower impact on blood sugar.

4. Portion Control:

- Pay attention to portion sizes to avoid overeating. Tailor daily caloric intake based on factors such as weight, activity level, and health goals. A dietitian can provide guidance on the appropriate amount of daily calories.

5. Lean Proteins:

- Include lean protein sources in the diet, such as poultry, lean pork, oily fish (like salmon and mackerel), and legumes. Protein aids in muscle maintenance and helps keep individuals feeling full.

6. Healthy Fats:

- Incorporate moderate amounts of healthy fats, including monounsaturated and polyunsaturated fats found in olive oil, avocados, nuts, and seeds. These fats support overall health without significantly impacting blood sugar levels.

7. Low-Fat Dairy:

- Include low-fat dairy options for essential nutrients like calcium and protein. These options contribute to bone health without excess saturated fat.

8. Limit Sugary Foods and Drinks:

- Minimize or eliminate sugary drinks, desserts, and other high-sugar foods. These can cause rapid spikes in blood sugar levels, making management more challenging.

9. Avoid Processed and High-Sodium Foods:

- Reduce intake of processed foods, especially those high in sodium. Opt for fresh, whole foods to better control sodium levels and support heart health.

10. Meal Timing:

- Pay attention to meal timing. Spreading meals and snacks throughout the day helps maintain steady blood sugar levels. Consistency in meal timing is beneficial for individuals on medication.

11. Hydration:

- Stay well-hydrated with water. Limit sugary drinks and caffeinated beverages, as they can potentially impact blood sugar levels.

12. Individualized Carbohydrate Counting:

- Some individuals benefit from carbohydrate counting, a method that involves tracking the amount of carbohydrates consumed at each meal. This can help with insulin management for those using insulin therapy.

13. Regular Monitoring:

- Monitor blood sugar levels regularly, especially after meals, to assess the impact of dietary choices. This information helps refine the dietary plan over time.

14. Continuous Learning:

- Stay informed about nutrition and diabetes management. Regularly consult with healthcare professionals to adapt the diet to changing health needs.

In essence, a diabetes-controlling diet involves a holistic and personalized approach. By focusing on whole, nutrient-dense foods, managing carbohydrates, and embracing a balanced and mindful approach to eating, individuals with diabetes can actively contribute to effective blood sugar control and overall well-being.

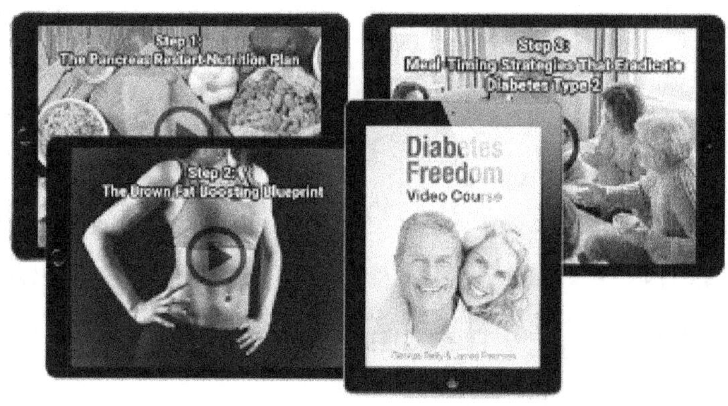

Click Here To Access Diabetes Diet Recipes

Exercise to Control Diabetes:

Exercise is a powerful tool in the management of diabetes, particularly type 2 diabetes. It offers a range of benefits that contribute to improved blood sugar control, increased insulin sensitivity, and overall well-being. Here's a detailed exploration of the role of exercise in controlling diabetes:

1. Brisk Movement and Its Impact:

   - Engaging in at least 150 minutes of brisk movement per week is a cornerstone of diabetes management. Brisk movement includes activities that get the heart rate up, such as brisk walking, cycling, dancing, or household chores. These activities help burn calories, improve cardiovascular health, and assist in regulating blood sugar levels.

2. Flexibility and Variety:

   - Incorporating a variety of exercises ensures a comprehensive approach to health. While aerobic activities are essential, flexibility exercises, such as yoga or Pilates, contribute to overall fitness. They can enhance mobility and reduce the risk of injuries, especially important for individuals with diabetes.

3. Strength Training for Muscle Health:

   - Regular strength training sessions, involving lifting weights or bodyweight exercises, play a crucial role. Building and maintaining muscle mass improves insulin sensitivity, helping the body use insulin more effectively. It also contributes to weight management and supports overall metabolic health.

4. Adaptability for Individual Preferences:

   - The key to sustained exercise is finding activities that individuals enjoy. This could be anything from swimming to gardening, as long as it involves movement. The goal is to make exercise a regular part of the routine, promoting consistency and long-term adherence.

5. Short Bursts for Busy Lifestyles:

- Studies show that even short bursts of activity, as little as 10 minutes at a time, can offer significant health benefits. This is particularly valuable for individuals with busy schedules, as it allows for flexibility in integrating exercise into daily life.

6. Consultation with Healthcare Providers:

- Before starting any exercise regimen, it's crucial to consult with healthcare providers, especially for those with existing health conditions. They can provide guidance on safe exercise levels, particularly for individuals on medications that may affect blood sugar or cardiovascular function.

7. Monitoring Blood Sugar Levels:

- Regular monitoring of blood sugar levels, especially before and after exercise, is essential. This helps individuals understand how different activities impact blood sugar and allows for adjustments in medication or dietary intake accordingly.

8. Integration into Daily Routine:

- Making exercise a seamless part of daily life contributes to its sustainability. This could involve taking the stairs instead of the elevator, walking short distances instead of driving, or incorporating physical activity into recreational pursuits.

9. Individualized Approach:

- Exercise plans should be individualized, considering factors such as fitness level, age, and overall health. This ensures that the chosen activities are safe and tailored to the individual's specific needs and goals.

10. Lifelong Commitment:

- Diabetes management through exercise is a lifelong commitment. As individuals age or their health status changes, adjustments to the exercise routine may be necessary. Regular check-ins with healthcare providers ensure that the exercise plan aligns with evolving health needs.

In conclusion, exercise is a dynamic and adaptable component of diabetes management. By embracing a variety of activities, incorporating regular strength training, and making exercise a personalized and enjoyable part of daily life, individuals with diabetes can harness its benefits for improved blood sugar control and overall well-being.

Lose Weight to Control Diabetes:

Losing weight is a significant and achievable goal in the management of diabetes, particularly type 2 diabetes. Weight loss can lead to improved insulin sensitivity, better blood sugar control, and a range of other health benefits. Here's a detailed exploration of the role of weight loss in controlling diabetes:

1. Gradual and Sustainable Approach:

   - The emphasis is on gradual and sustainable weight loss. Crash diets or extreme measures are generally discouraged, as they can be challenging to maintain and may not provide lasting results. Aiming for a modest and realistic weight loss goal, often as little as 5-10% of initial body weight, is associated with meaningful health improvements.

2. Caloric Balance and Portion Control:

   - Weight loss fundamentally involves creating a caloric deficit, where the calories burned exceed the calories consumed. Portion control is essential, focusing on mindful eating and recognizing hunger and fullness cues. Working with a dietitian can provide personalized guidance on appropriate caloric intake.

3. Whole Foods and Nutrient Density:

   - Prioritizing whole, nutrient-dense foods supports both weight loss and overall health. These foods, rich in vitamins, minerals, and fiber, contribute to satiety and help individuals feel full on fewer calories. The focus is on nourishing the body with quality nutrients.

4. Physical Activity for Weight Management:

   - Regular physical activity is integral to weight loss. Exercise not only burns calories but also helps build and preserve lean muscle mass, which is crucial for metabolic health. Combining aerobic activities with strength training contributes to an effective weight management strategy.

5. Individualized Plans:

   - Weight loss plans should be individualized, considering factors such as age, health status, and personal preferences. What works for one person may not be suitable for another. Collaborating with healthcare providers, including dietitians and fitness experts, ensures tailored and sustainable weight loss strategies.

6. Behavioral Changes and Mindful Eating:

   - Addressing the behavioral aspects of eating is essential. Mindful eating, recognizing emotional triggers for eating, and adopting healthy coping mechanisms contribute to long-term success. Behavioral changes are integral to breaking unhealthy patterns and establishing a positive relationship with food.

7. Regular Monitoring and Accountability:

   - Regular monitoring of progress and maintaining accountability are key components. This could involve keeping a food diary, tracking physical activity, or seeking support from healthcare providers, friends, or support groups. Celebrating small victories along the way reinforces positive behaviors.

8. Medical Supervision for Health Conditions:

- Individuals with diabetes often have other health conditions that may impact weight loss strategies. Medical supervision is crucial, especially for those on medications that may influence weight. Adjustments to medication or treatment plans may be necessary as weight loss progresses.

9. Long-Term Lifestyle Changes:

- The goal is not just to lose weight temporarily but to make lasting lifestyle changes. This includes adopting healthier eating habits, regular physical activity, and stress management techniques. Sustainable changes contribute to weight maintenance and ongoing diabetes control.

10. Improvements Beyond Blood Sugar Control:

- Weight loss brings about improvements beyond blood sugar control. It positively affects blood pressure, cholesterol levels, and cardiovascular health. It also reduces the risk of other obesity-related conditions, contributing to an overall enhancement of well-being.

In conclusion, losing weight is a multifaceted approach that goes beyond simply shedding pounds. It involves creating a sustainable caloric deficit, adopting healthier eating patterns, and incorporating regular physical activity. The journey is individualized, focusing on long-term changes that positively impact both weight and diabetes management.

Medication to Control Diabetes:

Controlling diabetes often involves a comprehensive approach, and for many individuals, medication is a crucial component. The choice of medication depends on various factors, including the type of diabetes, individual health history, and the effectiveness of lifestyle changes. Here's a detailed exploration of the role of medication in controlling diabetes:

1. Personalized Medication Plans:

   - Medication plans are highly personalized, reflecting the uniqueness of each individual's health profile. Diabetes medications aim to address specific aspects of blood sugar regulation, and the selection is based on factors such as the type of diabetes (type 1 or type 2), overall health, and the presence of any other medical conditions.

2. Oral Medications for Type 2 Diabetes:

- Individuals with type 2 diabetes often begin with oral medications. These medications work in various ways, such as improving insulin sensitivity, reducing glucose production by the liver, or enhancing insulin release from the pancreas. Common classes of oral medications include metformin, sulfonylureas, meglitinides, and thiazolidinediones.

3. Injectable Medications:

- In some cases, individuals with type 2 diabetes may need injectable medications. This includes GLP-1 receptor agonists and insulin. GLP-1 receptor agonists stimulate insulin release and reduce glucose production, while insulin may be required to manage blood sugar levels more directly.

4. Insulin Therapy for Type 1 Diabetes:

- Individuals with type 1 diabetes, where the body does not produce insulin, require insulin therapy. This is typically administered through injections or an insulin pump. Insulin therapy aims to mimic the natural insulin release in response to meals and regulate blood sugar levels throughout the day.

5. Combination Therapy:

- In some cases, a combination of medications may be prescribed to achieve optimal blood sugar control. This could involve combining oral medications, using a combination of oral medications and injectables, or combining different types of insulin.

6. Regular Monitoring and Adjustments:

   - Regular monitoring of blood sugar levels is essential for individuals on medication. This helps healthcare providers assess the effectiveness of the current regimen and make adjustments as needed. Dosage adjustments, changes in medication, or additions to the treatment plan may be recommended based on ongoing monitoring.

7. Trial and Error:

   - Finding the most effective medication or combination often involves a degree of trial and error. Individuals may need to try different medications or dosages to achieve the desired blood sugar control. Regular communication with healthcare providers is crucial during this process.

8. Consideration of Other Health Conditions:

   - Medication plans take into account other health conditions that may coexist with diabetes. For example, individuals with diabetes and hypertension may be prescribed medications that address both conditions simultaneously.

9. Lifestyle Changes and Medication Synergy:

- Medication is often complemented by lifestyle changes. Adopting a healthy diet, regular exercise, and weight management can enhance the effectiveness of medications. Some individuals may find that as they make positive lifestyle changes, the need for medication may decrease.

10. Regular Follow-Ups and Adherence:

- Regular follow-ups with healthcare providers are crucial to monitor progress and address any concerns. Adherence to the prescribed medication plan is essential for effective blood sugar control. Open communication about any challenges or side effects helps healthcare providers make necessary adjustments.

In conclusion, medication plays a vital role in diabetes management, working in conjunction with lifestyle changes. The goal is to achieve and maintain optimal blood sugar control, preventing complications and promoting overall well-being. Personalized medication plans, regular monitoring, and collaboration with healthcare providers are key elements in successful diabetes management.

Monitoring Blood Sugar:

Monitoring blood sugar is a fundamental aspect of diabetes management, providing valuable insights into how the body responds to various factors such as diet, exercise, and medication. Here's a detailed exploration of the importance and process of monitoring blood sugar:

1. Frequency of Monitoring:

- The frequency of blood sugar monitoring varies based on the type of diabetes, the individual's treatment plan, and overall health. Individuals with type 1 diabetes or those on insulin therapy often need to check their blood sugar multiple times a day. Those with type 2 diabetes may have a less frequent monitoring schedule, depending on their treatment regimen.

2. Blood Sugar Targets:

- Healthcare providers set individualized blood sugar targets based on factors like age, overall health, and the type and severity of diabetes. Common targets include fasting blood sugar levels and post-meal levels. For instance, the American Diabetes Association recommends a target range of 80 to 130 mg/dL before meals and less than 180 mg/dL two hours after meals.

3. Devices for Monitoring:

- Glucose meters, also known as glucometers, are commonly used for blood sugar monitoring. These portable devices provide a quick and accurate measure of blood sugar levels. Continuous glucose monitoring (CGM) systems are another option, offering real-time data and trends over time. Choosing the right device often depends on individual preferences, lifestyle, and treatment plan.

4. Monitoring Before and After Meals:

- Regular blood sugar checks before and after meals offer insights into how different foods impact blood sugar levels. This information helps individuals make informed choices about their diet and medication timing. Pre-meal monitoring provides a baseline, while post-meal monitoring reflects the body's response to food.

5. Integration with Lifestyle Factors:

- Monitoring blood sugar is not isolated; it's integrated with various lifestyle factors. Individuals track their blood sugar in relation to meals, physical activity, medication, and stress levels. This holistic approach helps identify patterns and triggers that influcncc blood sugar control.

6. Adjustments to Medication and Diet:

- Blood sugar readings guide adjustments to medication dosages and dietary choices. For instance, if post-meal readings consistently exceed the target range, healthcare providers may recommend changes to medication timing or dosage. Similarly, individuals can modify their diet based on how certain foods affect their blood sugar levels.

7. Regular Check-Ins with Healthcare Providers:

- Regular check-ins with healthcare providers are essential to review blood sugar data and make necessary adjustments to the treatment plan. These appointments provide an opportunity to discuss challenges, address concerns, and ensure that the current management strategy aligns with overall health goals.

8. Self-Empowerment and Awareness:

- Monitoring blood sugar fosters self-empowerment and awareness. Individuals gain a deeper understanding of their body's response to different factors, allowing them to take an active role in their diabetes management. This awareness extends beyond numerical readings to an overall understanding of how lifestyle choices impact health.

9. Recording and Analyzing Data:

- Keeping a record of blood sugar readings, along with notes about meals, physical activity, and medication, is valuable. This data becomes a powerful tool during healthcare provider consultations, facilitating a collaborative approach to diabetes management. Analyzing trends helps identify areas for improvement.

10. Education and Training:

- Proper education and training in using glucose monitoring devices are crucial. Individuals learn techniques for obtaining accurate readings, understanding the significance of different values, and troubleshooting common issues. Education empowers individuals to confidently manage their diabetes through effective monitoring.

In conclusion, monitoring blood sugar is a dynamic and personalized process that goes beyond numerical values. It's a tool for self-awareness, a guide for lifestyle choices, and a collaborative platform for healthcare providers and individuals to work together toward optimal diabetes management. Regular monitoring is not just about numbers; it's about fostering a deeper connection with one's health.

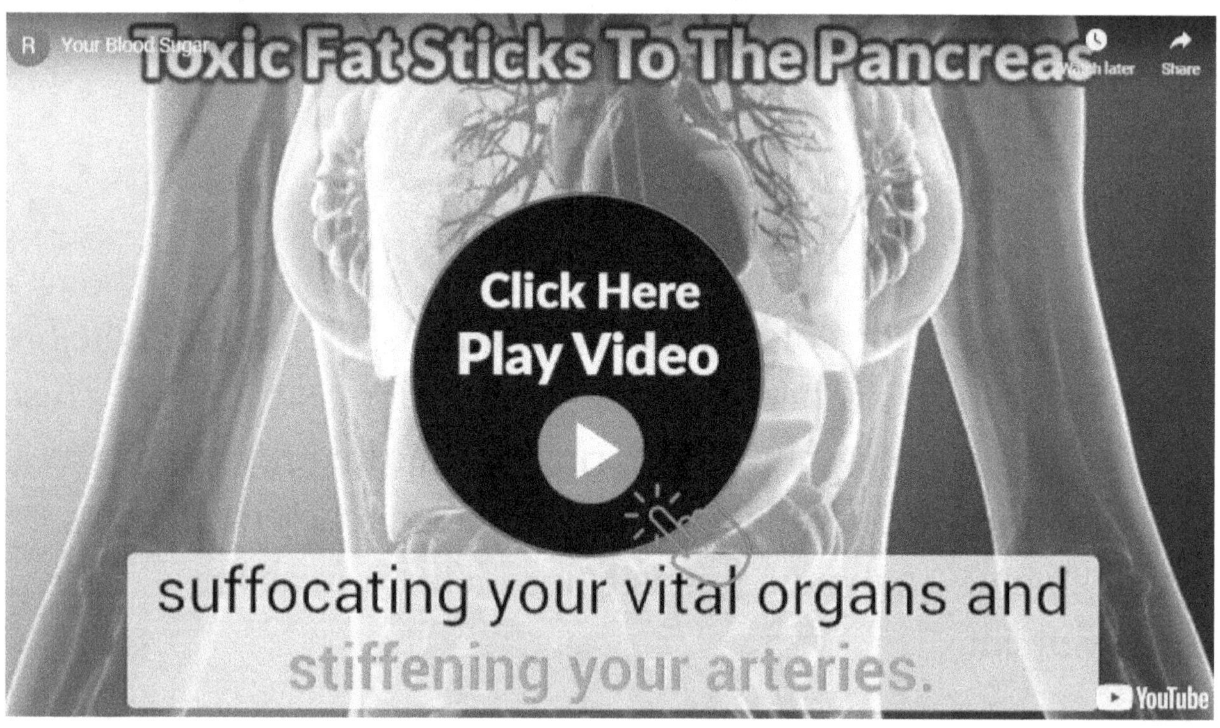

Watch: How Type 2 Diabetes Can Be Reverse?

Bariatric Surgery in Diabetes Management: -

Bariatric surgery, a surgical procedure designed to promote weight loss, has emerged as a significant intervention in the management of diabetes, particularly in cases where other methods have not achieved desired results. Here's a detailed exploration of bariatric surgery and its role in diabetes management:

1. Indications for Bariatric Surgery:

   - Bariatric surgery is considered for individuals with a body mass index (BMI) over 35, especially if they have obesity-related complications such as type 2 diabetes. In some cases, individuals with a BMI over 40 may be candidates for surgery, even in the absence of obesity-related complications.

2. Mechanisms of Action:

   - Bariatric surgery works through various mechanisms, with weight loss being a primary factor. Procedures such as gastric bypass, sleeve gastrectomy, and gastric banding reduce the size of the stomach, limiting food intake. Additionally, these surgeries can affect gut hormones, leading to improved insulin sensitivity and glucose metabolism.

3. Impact on Type 2 Diabetes:

- One of the notable outcomes of bariatric surgery is its impact on type 2 diabetes. Many individuals experience significant improvements in blood sugar control post-surgery, with some achieving remission. The surgery's effects on hormones and metabolic pathways contribute to enhanced insulin sensitivity and reduced glucose levels.

4. Weight Loss and Metabolic Changes:

- Bariatric surgery often results in substantial weight loss within the first year following the procedure. This weight loss is accompanied by metabolic changes that extend beyond the reduction in food intake. Hormonal alterations contribute to improvements in glucose regulation, lipid profiles, and overall metabolic health.

5. Timing and Considerations:

- The timing of bariatric surgery in the context of diabetes management is a crucial consideration. Some individuals may opt for surgery soon after a diabetes diagnosis, while others may explore it as a potential option after struggling with other interventions. Collaborative discussions with healthcare providers help individuals make informed decisions.

6. Selection of Surgical Procedure:

- Different types of bariatric surgeries are available, and the choice depends on individual health factors, preferences, and the desired outcomes. Gastric bypass, sleeve gastrectomy, and gastric banding are among the common procedures. Each has unique effects on weight loss and metabolic changes.

7. Multidisciplinary Approach:

- Bariatric surgery involves a multidisciplinary approach. Before the surgery, individuals typically undergo thorough evaluations, including psychological assessments and nutritional counseling. Post-surgery, ongoing support from healthcare providers, dietitians, and mental health professionals is crucial for long-term success.

8. Consideration of Comorbidities:

- Bariatric surgery is often considered not only for weight loss but also to address comorbidities such as diabetes, hypertension, and sleep apnea. The surgery's potential to improve or resolve these conditions contributes to its overall impact on individuals' health.

9. Lifestyle Changes Post-Surgery:

- Bariatric surgery is a catalyst for significant lifestyle changes. Individuals must adhere to specific dietary guidelines, adopt regular physical activity, and make behavioral adjustments to support the surgical outcomes. Post-surgery, ongoing lifestyle modifications are integral to maintaining weight loss and diabetes improvements.

10. Potential Risks and Considerations:

- While bariatric surgery has shown significant benefits, it's not without risks. Complications, although rare, can occur. Potential risks include infection, blood clots, and nutritional deficiencies. Individuals considering surgery should thoroughly discuss potential risks and benefits with their healthcare team.

In conclusion, bariatric surgery represents a transformative approach to diabetes management for individuals with obesity. Its impact extends beyond weight loss, encompassing metabolic improvements and, in some cases, diabetes remission. However, it requires a comprehensive and collaborative effort, involving healthcare professionals and individuals committed to making sustained lifestyle changes for long-term success.

Diabetes Complications to Watch Out For:

Managing diabetes requires vigilance not only in controlling blood sugar levels but also in monitoring and addressing potential complications. Here's a detailed exploration of the complications associated with diabetes that individuals need to be vigilant about:

1. Vision Problems:

- **Overview:** High blood sugar levels can damage the delicate blood vessels in the eyes, leading to vision problems.

 - **Complications:** Blurry vision is an early sign, and if left untreated, it may progress to permanent vision impairment or blindness.

 - **Preventive Measures:** Regular eye exams, keeping blood sugar, blood pressure, and cholesterol within normal ranges, and quitting smoking can reduce the risk.

2. Slow-Healing Wounds:

 - **Overview:** High blood sugar damages blood vessels, affecting circulation, and slowing down the healing of wounds, especially in the legs and feet.

 - **.Complications:** Reduced sensation in extremities (peripheral neuropathy) can lead to unnoticed injuries, increasing the risk of infections and, in severe cases, amputation.

 - **Preventive Measures:** Daily foot care, prompt attention to any injuries, and regular visits to a podiatrist can help prevent complications.

3. Heart Disease and Stroke:

 - **Overview:** Individuals with diabetes are at a highcr risk of heart disease and stroke compared to those without diabetes.

 - **.Complications:** Increased likelihood of heart attacks and strokes, leading causes of mortality in people with diabetes.

 - **.Preventive Measures:** Maintaining blood sugar within normal ranges, controlling blood pressure and cholesterol, adopting a healthy lifestyle, and quitting smoking are vital for heart health.

4. Kidney Disease (Nephropathy):

- **.Overview:** Prolonged high blood sugar can damage the kidneys over time, leading to kidney disease.

- **.Complications:** Impaired kidney function, potentially progressing to kidney failure, necessitating dialysis or transplantation.

- **.Preventive Measures:** Monitoring blood pressure, maintaining tight control over blood sugar levels, and regular kidney function tests are crucial for early detection and management.

5. .Nerve Damage (Neuropathy):

- **.Overview:** Elevated blood sugar levels can damage nerves throughout the body, causing neuropathy.

- **.Complications:** Symptoms include pain, tingling, or numbness in extremities, and it can lead to problems with digestion, sexual function, and coordination.

- **.Preventive Measures:** Tight blood sugar control, regular monitoring, and lifestyle changes can help prevent or manage neuropathic complications.

6. .Cardiovascular Autonomic Neuropathy (CAN):

- .**Overview:** Diabetes can affect the nerves that control the heart, leading to cardiovascular autonomic neuropathy.

- .**Complications:** Increased risk of heart rhythm abnormalities, fainting, and sudden cardiac death.

- .**Preventive Measures:** Managing diabetes effectively, adopting heart-healthy lifestyle choices, and regular cardiovascular monitoring.

7. .Peripheral Arterial Disease (PAD):

- .**Overview:** Diabetes contributes to the hardening of arteries, limiting blood flow to the extremities.

- .**Complications**: PAD can lead to leg pain, ulcers, and an increased risk of infections and amputations.

- .**Preventive Measures:** Maintaining a healthy lifestyle, including regular exercise, and controlling blood sugar, blood pressure, and cholesterol.

8. .Skin Complications:

- .**Overview:** Diabetes can affect the skin, leading to various complications, including infections and conditions like acanthosis nigricans.

- .**Complications:** Increased susceptibility to bacterial and fungal infections, poor wound healing, and skin changes.

- **.Preventive Measures:** Good hygiene practices, regular skin checks, and prompt treatment of any skin issues can help prevent complications.

9. .Hypoglycemia and Hyperglycemia:

- **.Overview:** Fluctuations in blood sugar levels, both low (hypoglycemia) and high (hyperglycemia), can pose immediate health risks.

- **.Complications:** Hypoglycemia can lead to seizures or unconsciousness, while persistent hyperglycemia can contribute to long-term complications.

- **.Preventive Measures**: Regular monitoring, timely adjustments to medication, and adherence to a diabetes management plan can help maintain stable blood sugar levels.

10. .Mental Health:

- **.Overview:** Diabetes can impact mental health, contributing to conditions like depression and diabetes distress.

- **.Complications:** Untreated mental health issues can negatively affect diabetes management and overall well-being.

- **.Preventive Measures:** Regular mental health check-ins, seeking support when needed, and adopting stress management strategies are essential components of comprehensive diabetes care.

In conclusion, individuals with diabetes need to be proactive in monitoring their health, addressing potential complications promptly, and adopting a holistic approach to diabetes management that encompasses both physical and mental well-being. Regular communication with healthcare providers and a commitment to a healthy lifestyle are integral to preventing and managing diabetes-related complications.

.Conclusion: Taking Charge of Your Diabetes Journey:

In the intricate landscape of diabetes management, the journey is multifaceted, requiring dedication, awareness, and a proactive approach. Here's a nuanced exploration of the conclusion drawn from the comprehensive information provided:

1. .Seriousness of Type 2 Diabetes:

- Recognizing type 2 diabetes as a serious condition is the first step in the journey. Understanding its prevalence, potential complications, and impact on various aspects of health underscores the importance of proactive management.

2. .Empowerment through Education:

- Education becomes a cornerstone in the quest for effective diabetes management. Seeking knowledge about the condition, its risk factors, and the diverse strategies for control empowers individuals to make informed decisions about their health.

3. .Early Intervention and Prediabetes Awareness:

- Emphasizing the significance of early intervention, particularly during the prediabetes stage, highlights the potential for reversing the course of the condition. Awareness and lifestyle changes at this juncture can be transformative in preventing the progression to full diabetes.

4. .Personalized Diabetes Screening:

- Diabetes diagnosis hinges on proactive and personalized screening, especially for individuals with specific risk factors. Regular blood sugar tests, A1C measurements, and urine tests provide a comprehensive overview, enabling timely intervention.

5. .Lifestyle Changes as the Foundation:

- The bedrock of diabetes management lies in lifestyle modifications. Cultivating a healthy diet, regular physical activity, and weight management are pivotal in controlling blood sugar levels and fostering overall well-being.

6. .Dietary Guidelines for Diabetes Control:

- The dietary landscape for diabetes control is intricate but navigable. Tailoring dietary choices to individual needs, focusing on whole foods, and being mindful of carbohydrate intake form the essence of a diabetes-friendly diet. The symbiotic relationship between a diabetes diet and overall family health underscores the universality of these principles.

7. .Exercise as a Diabetes Ally:

- Exercise emerges as a powerful ally in diabetes control. From brisk walking to strength training, physical activity not only aids in blood sugar regulation but also contributes to weight management and cardiovascular health.

8. .Weight Loss as a Gradual Transformation:

- Weight loss, if necessary, need not be drastic. A gradual and sustainable approach, supported by lifestyle changes, can yield significant benefits in diabetes management. Small, consistent steps can pave the way for lasting improvements.

9. .Medication and Individualized Plans:

- Acknowledging the role of medication in diabetes control brings forth the concept of individualized plans. Collaborating with healthcare providers, understanding medication options, and being open to adjustments create a dynamic framework for success.

10. .Vigilance through Blood Sugar Monitoring:

- Regular blood sugar monitoring is not merely a task; it is a tool for self-empowerment and awareness. Understanding the nuances of testing, interpreting results, and integrating this information with lifestyle factors forms a holistic approach to diabetes control.

11. .Bariatric Surgery as a Transformative Option:

- Bariatric surgery, while not a one-size-fits-all solution, stands as a transformative option for those struggling with obesity-related diabetes. The decision involves a thorough exploration of benefits, risks, and a commitment to post-surgery lifestyle changes.

12. .Complications: A Call for Vigilance:

- The mention of potential complications serves as a clarion call for vigilance. From vision problems to cardiovascular issues, staying proactive in preventive measures and early intervention becomes paramount in the diabetes journey.

13. .Mental Health as an Integral Component:

- Recognizing the impact of diabetes on mental health underscores the holistic nature of the journey. Addressing mental health concerns, seeking support, and embracing stress management contribute to overall well-being.

14. .Empowering Self-Management:

- The journey with diabetes is a dynamic interplay between healthcare professionals and individuals. Self-management becomes a central theme, emphasizing the role of the individual in making daily choices that influence long-term health.

15. .Never Too Late for Positive Changes:

- The conclusion resonates with the powerful message that positive changes are never too late. Even amidst the challenges of diabetes, the smallest adjustments in lifestyle, diet, and mindset can pave the way for significant improvements.

In essence, the conclusion of the diabetes journey is a call to action—a call to embrace education, make informed choices, and embark on a path where proactive management becomes a way of life. The journey is a continuum, with each step contributing to a healthier, more empowered future.

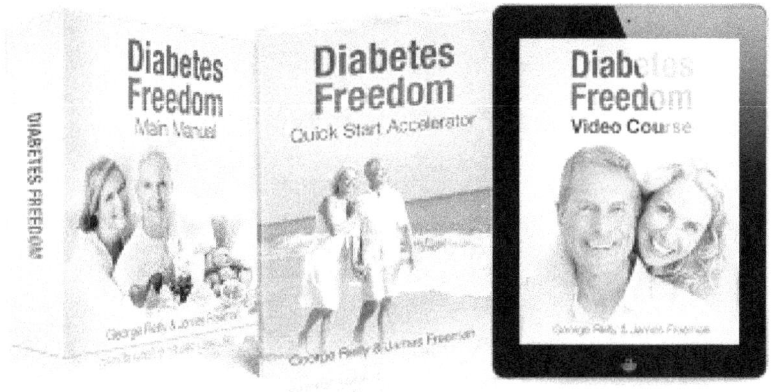

Click Here To Get Freedom From Diabetes Type 1 & Type 2